# Pregnancy Nutrition

*Pregnancy Food Pregnancy Recipes*

*Healthy Pregnancy Diet Pregnancy*

*Health Pregnancy Eating and Recipes*

*Nutritional Tips And*

*63 Delicious Recipes for Moms-to-Be*

By Corinne Watson and John McArthur

# COPYRIGHT

The author and publisher are not responsible for the use, effectiveness or safety of any procedure or treatment mentioned in this book. The publisher is not responsible for errors and omissions.

**Warning**

All treatment of any medical condition (without exception) must always be done under supervision of a qualified medical professional. The fact that a substance is "natural" does not necessarily mean that it has no side effects or interaction with other medications.

Medical professionals are qualified and experienced to give advice on side effects and interactions of all types of medication.

# Table of Contents

## Scrumptious Lunches ......................................................... 90

# HEALTHY EATING DURING PREGNANCY

Nothing sheds light on your diet choices like knowing you have a growing baby inside of you. All at once you become more aware of your diet as you start to focus on the health of your precious growing bundle. Making sure that you are eating a healthy balanced diet during pregnancy is crucial. Your nutritional needs differ and the amount of calories that you need on a daily basis changes.

Making good diet choices is important for your health and the health of your baby. You need to make sure that you are getting the extra calories that you need by eating a nutritious balanced diet as opposed to a diet filled with high-calorie junk food. Of course it goes without saying that you also need to treat yourself to some of your favorite foods from time to time.

You will find that during your pregnancy you will have to contend with cravings and increased hunger. Making wise diet choices is very hard when you are that hungry! That is why it helps to have a plan and some easy and healthy recipes on hand! Let's take a closer look at what your diet should look like during pregnancy. There are certain foods that you will need to avoid and others that you will need to eat to ensure you are getting all the nutrients your body needs to support your growing baby.

## FOODS TO AVOID

- There are certain foods that contain bacteria that could harm your unborn baby and it is best for you to avoid them. Here is a list of the foods and drinks that should either be avoided, or consumed in moderation.
- Stay away from seafood that might be raw, contaminated or slightly undercooked.
- Don't eat raw fish or shellfish like oysters and clams.
- Avoid seafood that is high in mercury. Too much mercury in your diet could negatively affect the development of your baby's nervous system. Specific fish to avoid include Tilefish, King Mackerel, Shark and Swordfish.
- Avoid drinking milk that has not been pasteurized and eating soft cheeses like Camembert, Brie and Blue Cheese.
- Make sure that you don't consume any undercooked meat, eggs, or poultry as these could cause bacterial food poisoning.
- Avoid eating fruits and vegetables that have not been washed properly as they could contain harmful bacteria.

- Avoid drinking too much caffeine as it has been shown to have an effect on your baby's heart rate if consumed excessively. You should try and have no more than 200 milligrams per day. One cup of coffee contains about 95 milligrams of caffeine. If there is any way that you could completely avoid caffeine that would be best.

- Alcohol should be completely avoided during pregnancy. A very small amount is not likely to affect your baby but even small amounts have not been proven safe to an unborn baby. Large amounts of alcohol could cause Fetal Alcohol Syndrome, which could result in low birth weight, heart problems, facial deformities and mental retardation.

## A BALANCED DIET

You have it within your power to give your baby the best possible start in life, just by ensuring that your diet is balanced and full of nutrients. A good diet can go a long way in minimizing complications like anemia and pre-eclampsia and even in reducing the severity of pregnancy symptoms such as morning sickness, fatigue, constipation etc. Eating a good sensible diet will also help you return to your original weight without too much of a struggle.

The best thing you can do to ensure your body and is getting all the nutrition it needs to support your growing baby is to eat a balanced diet. You need a little of everything every day.  You should eat a selection of foods from the four main food groups which are starchy foods, foods rich in protein, dairy products and fruits and vegetable.  Here is an indication of how much body needs from the different food groups on a daily basis:

**Protein:**

Ideally, you should eat three servings of protein every day. Remember that protein is also found in milk, cheese, yoghurt and other food substances that contain a lot of calcium.

**Fruits and Vegetables:**

Aim to eat 5 servings of fruits and vegetables daily. Three of those servings should come from yellow fruits as well as yellow and green leafy vegetables such as broccoli, carrots, winter squash, sweet potato, pumpkin, and mangoes. These are packed with vitamin A that is in the form of beta-carotene. Your baby needs this to help with the growth of his/her cells, bones, skin and eyes. Your last two servings can come from the other types of fruits and vegetables like bananas, apples, grapes, peaches, mushrooms, green beans, potatoes etc;. Most of these are rich in minerals such as potassium, magnesium and phytochemicals.

### Foods rich in Iron:

Foods like beef, liver, spinach, cooked legumes, sardines and all Soya products are rich in iron. You need an extra supply of iron for your baby's developing blood supply and for your blood supply, which doubles during pregnancy. You will need to take an iron supplement from your 20th week, since you probably won't get enough just from your diet. Most women take an extra 30 to 50 mg – this is in addition to what they are already getting from a pregnancy supplement.

### Foods high in salt:

It is never good to consume too much salt whether you are pregnant or not. Be sure to eat salty foods in moderation, especially while you are pregnant. If you were previously addicted to pickles and potato chips, now is the time to replace those foods with a healthier alternative. It was once thought that pregnant women should drastically reduce their intake of salt but now it is widely accepted that it is important for pregnant women to eat some salt. Salt is necessary to maintain sufficient levels of fluid in the body.

## Water and other fluids:

You are not eating for two, but you are certainly drinking for two! You and your growing baby need extra fluids during pregnancy. If you are in the habit of drinking hardly anything during the day now is the time to change that. You need water to help with yours and your baby's kidney and liver function and to aid in the flushing of toxins from your body. Adequate fluid will also help with constipation, the prevention of UTI's, fatigue and will promote a good milk supply later on.  An added bonus is that your skin will be nice and soft and your general complexion will be better. Aim to drink about 8 250 ml glasses of water a day. Remember that some of your fluid could also come from soup, fruit drinks, milk and sugar-free soft drinks. Just try and make sure that most of it comes from water.

## Carbohydrates:

There are so many great complex carbohydrates that you can and should eat while pregnancy like whole wheat bread, brown rice, oatmeal, and whole grain pastas and tortillas. Try and stay away from refined grains which are cereals and breads which have been made using white flour. There is so much goodness in the whole grain variety of most foods that it is always the better option. You can eat as much as 9 whole grain servings each day. A typical serving would be a slice of whole grain bread or 1/2 cup whole grain rice or pasta.  These foods are packed with fiber, minerals and B vitamins which are needed for the development and growth of your baby's body.

## Foods Rich in Calcium:

While pregnant you will need at least 1200 milligrams of calcium daily. This could come from milk, cottage cheese, yoghurt, orange juice, broccoli, greens, or sardines to name a few.

## Fatty Foods:

It might surprise you to know that you actually need a certain amount of fats in your diet every day.  It would actually be dangerous to you and your baby if you decided to completely eliminate fat from your diet. Because so many people have suffered the consequences of too much fat in their diet, we often want to run in the opposite direction when we see any fatty food. You will be pleased to know that 20 to 30% of your daily calorie intake should come from fats. It is important for you not to exceed this amount if you don't want to gain excess weight during your pregnancy. Remember that some healthy foods like whole grains and calcium foods also contain fat that should be taken into account and aim to eat more unsaturated fats found in nuts, fish and flaxseed.

# Breakfast At Its Best

## Omelet with Crab and Snow Pea Filling

### Ingredients

40 g 2-minute noodles

2 tbsp Cheese

1.10 oz (30g) finely sliced and trimmed snow peas

6 oz (170g) can crab meat (remove excess liquid)

1/4 small sliced red capsicum

0.70 oz (20g) snow pea sprouts

2 eggs

1 tsp butter

2 slices of toasted multigrain bread

### Preparation

Start by cooking your 2 minute noodles according to package instructions. In a separate bowl whisk the 2 eggs. Now stir the cooked noodles and cheese into the egg mixture. Season with salt and pepper to taste.

Put a dollop of butter into a non-stick frying pan. Once it has heated slowly pour the egg mixture into the pan. Reduce the heat and allow to cook for 5 minutes, or until the bottom of the omelet has browned.

Sprinkle the trimmed snow peas, capsicum and crab meat over half of the omelet and fold over to cover ingredients.

Remove the omelet from the pan and carefully plate it.

Scatter the snow pea sprouts over the omelet to add the last finishing touch. Serve with bread. Serves 1

# FRESH HERB OMELET

## Ingredients

3 free-range eggs

1/2 tsp extra virgin olive oil

2 tbsp finely shredded fresh herbs: Parsley, basil, chives, parsley, and marjoram

Salt and Pepper

1 tsp unsalted butter

Wholewheat bread

## Preparation

In a medium sized bowl, whisk the eggs and season with salt and pepper.

Heat the butter and oil in a frying pan. Once it starts to sizzle, pour in the egg mixture. As the bottom of the omelet starts to cook, lift it on one side and allow the uncooked egg to run underneath it. Keep doing this until the omelet is cooked all the way through.

Top one side of the cooked omelet with the shredded herbs and fold over. Carefully remove the omelet from the pan and plate. Serve with toasted wholewheat bread.

## CHEESE AND ASPARAGUS OMELET

### Ingredients

½ cup egg substitute

4 spears of asparagus

Nonstick cooking spray

½ tsp. olive oil

¼ tsp. ground black pepper

1 fat-free or low fat cheese wedge cut into pieces

1 tbsp. sweet red peppers

1 tsp. chopped parsley

### Preparation

Lightly coat an unheated large nonstick skillet with cooking spray. Add asparagus to skillet and pan-roast over medium-high heat for 7 minutes or until browned and crisp-tender, turning occasionally. Set aside.

In a medium bowl combine egg whites and pepper. Using a fork, beat until combined but not frothy. In an 8-inch nonstick skillet heat oil over medium-high heat. Add egg whites to skillet. Reduce heat to medium. As eggs start to set, use a heatproof silicone spatula to gently lift edges of set egg white, tilting pan to allow liquid egg white to run under set egg. Continue until egg is set but still shiny.

Arrange the asparagus spears on half of the eggs in skillet. Top evenly with cheese. Fold the unfilled half of the eggs over the asparagus and cheese. Gently slide the omelet out of the skillet onto a serving plate. Sprinkle omelet with red sweet pepper slivers and parsley. Makes 1 (1 omelet) serving.

# ENGLISH MUFFIN TOPPED WITH SAUSAGE, TOMATO AND CHEESE

## Ingredients

1 whole grain English muffin

1 turkey or vegetable sausage patty

1 slice reduced fat cheese

## Preparation

Toast the English muffin and heat your sausage at the same time.

Place the heated sausage onto your muffin and top with the slice of cheese. It's that easy!

## GUILT-FREE BREAKFAST PIZZA

### Ingredients

1 whole wheat thin pizza base

¼ cup cheese

2 tbs pizza sauce

1 tbsp of chopped green pepper

1 tbsp fresh basil

### Preparation

Spread the pizza sauce on the base and then add the basil, cheese, green pepper, and basil.

Place in the microwave for 1 min until the cheese has melted.

# Crispy Hotcakes topped with Yoghurt and Blueberries

## Ingredients

1 3/4 cup self-raising flour (wholemeal)

1 cup fresh blueberries

3 cups fat free yoghurt

1/2 cup apple sauce

1 tsp vanilla extract

1 separated egg

Egg whites from 2 eggs

## Preparation

Beat the egg whites together until you see soft peaks have formed.

In a medium sized bowl combine the flour, 1/2 of the blueberries, vanilla extract, apple sauce, and 2 cups of the yoghurt. Once properly combined, fold in the egg whites.

Heat oil in a frying pan and use 1/4 cup of the batter for one hotcake. When frying, only turn once bubbles have started forming on the surface. They should be golden brown and cooked through.

Once cooked, top each hotcake with some of the remaining blueberries and yogurt. Serves 6.

# Delicious Oats topped with Bananas and Walnuts

## Ingredients

1 1/3 cup rolled oats

2 cups water

1 cup low-fat milk

2 thickly sliced medium sized bananas

1/2 cup chopped walnuts

1 tbsp honey

1 additional cup low-fat milk (for use on cooked oats – optional)

## Preparation

Pour the water and the milk (1 cup) into a pot and bring to the boil.

Lower the heat and add oats. Allow to simmer for about 5 min. Oats should be soft and creamy when ready.

Put oats in bowls and top with honey, walnuts and banana sliced. Add extra milk if desired. Serves 4.

# Rye Bread topped with Corn, Ricotta and Spinach

## Ingredients

1 can corn kernels (drained)

1/2 cup chopped spinach leaves

2 tbsp low-fat ricotta cheese

1 slices toasted rye bread

## Preparation

Place drained corn in microwaveable bowl and heat on high for 30 seconds.

Stir ricotta cheese and spinach into corn.

Place rye bread on plate and top each slice with the corn, cheese and spinach combination.

# Wholesome Homemade Berry Muesli

## Ingredients

1 cup rolled oats

1/2 cup all-bran

1/4 cup dried cranberries

2 cups low-fat milk

1 sliced large banana

1/2 cup juicy fresh raspberries

## Preparation

Mix the rolled oats, all bran and cranberries to make your muesli.

Place muesli in bowls and finish off by topping with raspberries, milk and banana slices. Guaranteed to be crispy and delicious!

# Nutritious Dinner Recipes

## Peri-Peri Pork Cutlets with Gaucamole

### Ingredients

4 pork cutlets without the rind

1 tbsp olive oil

Leaves of 1 small romaine lettuce

1/2 cup peri-peri marinade

1 lime, halved

Guacamole

1 Avocado Pear

1/4 cup shredded coriander leaves

### Preparation

Beat the pork with a meat mallet to flatten in. It should be 2cm thick when you are done. Now drench the cutlets in marinade and allow them to stand for at least 5 minutes.

To make the guacamole mash the avocado flesh and combine with the coriander leaves. Add salt and pepper to taste.

In a separate bowl toss the Romaine lettuce with 1/2 the olive oil and season.

Once you have heated oil in a pan, cook the pork for 5 minutes, turning only once. Cook longer if you desire.

Serve cooked pork with Romaine lettuce, lime halves and guacamole. Serves 4.

## Curry Infused Beef Pilaf

### Ingredients

14 oz (400g) lean beef mince

1 1/2 tbsp olive oil

3 finely chopped green onions

8.8 oz (250g) cherry tomatoes

1 cup rinsed basmati rice

2 1/2 cups chicken stock (reduced salt)

1 tbsp curry powder

1/2 cup flat-leaf parsley leaves

1 tsp ground cumin

1 tsp ground cinnamon

1/4 cup currants

### Preparation

Preheat oven to 365°F (180°C). Now lay cherry tomatoes on a baking tray on some baking paper. Pour 2 teaspoons of oil over the tomatoes and season with salt and pepper. Place in oven for 20 minutes until tomatoes become soft.

Place a saucepan on the stove on medium heat and add remaining oil. Add the cumin, cinnamon, curry powder and mince to heated oil and allow to cook while stirring for 4 minutes. Add rice.

Pour the chicken stock into the rice dish and bring to the boil. Now pour the mixture into a large oven dish. Cover and bake for approximately 25 minutes, or until all the liquid has been soaked into the rice.

To add the finishing touches, stir the tomatoes, currants and green onions into the dish. Allow to stand for a few minutes before serving. Add parsley just before dishing up. Serves 4

# CREAMY SNOW PEA CHICKEN AND TOMATO PASTA

## Ingredients

17.6 oz (500g) chicken breast fillets

12.35 oz (350g) penne pasta

3.5 oz (100g) trimmed and halved snow peas

1 tsp olive oil

1 x (17.6 oz) 500g Tomato Basil Pasta Sauce

## Preparation

Cook pasta according to package instructions until al dente. 30 seconds before the pasta is ready stir in the snow peas. Drain the pasta and place back into pot.

Heat some oil in a large frying pan. Season chicken to taste and then fry for a few minutes until the chicken is cooked all the way through. Once cooked remove from the pan and allow to stand for a few minutes.

Pour Tomato Basil Pasta Sauce into your pasta and heat over medium heat. Once properly heated add thinly sliced chicken pieces and combine. Dinner is served! Serves 4.

## Chicken and Sun-dried Tomato Pasta

### Ingredients

10.6 oz (300g) chicken breast fillet slices

14.10 oz (400g) fettuccine pasta

2 tsp olive oil

12.7 fl. oz. (375ml) evaporated milk

1.7 oz (50g) baby spinach

2 shredded green onions

1/2 cup chopped sun-dried tomatoes

1/4 cup pitted black olives

1 tbsp corn flour

Wholewheat Bread

### Preparation

Cook pasta according to package directions until al Dente. Once cooked, drain and place back into the pot that you cooked it in.

While the pasta is cooking, heat some oil in a pan. Fry onions until brown before adding chicken pieces. Continue to cook for another

3 minutes or until chicken is cooked the way you like it. Now add the black olives and tomatoes. Toss.

In a jug combine the corn flour with 1 tbsp of cold water and stir to form a paste before stirring in the evaporated milk.

Pour the mixture over the chicken in the frying pan and allow to cook for 2 minutes until the sauce thickens. Season as desired.

Add the contents of the frying pan to the cooked pasta and toss in the baby spinach.  Allow to cook over low heat for a few minutes. Serve with buttered whole-wheat bread.  Serves 4.

# Chicken Pasta with Cherry Tomatoes

## Ingredients

13.2 oz (375g) uncooked spaghetti

2 17.6 oz (500g) chicken breast fillets

8.8oz (250g) cherry tomatoes

1 finely chopped brown onion

1/2 cup grated parmesan cheese

2 finely shredded garlic cloves

1 tbsp olive oil

12.7 fl. oz (375ml) can Light Evaporated Milk

2 tsp fresh thyme leaves

2 tbsp chopped fresh chives

3.5 oz (100g) baby spinach

## Preparation

Cook spaghetti according to package instructions. Once cooked, drain it and put it back into the pot.

While the spaghetti is cooking heat half the oil in a frying pan. Once the oil is heated fry the chicken the breasts for around 6 minutes per side until thoroughly cooked and slightly browned. Remove the cooked chicken from the pan and slice into thin slices on chopping board.

Heat the remaining oil and sauté the onion and garlic. After a few minutes add the tomatoes and allow to continue cooking until they have softened.

Pour in the evaporated milk, stir in the chives and thyme and season with salt and pepper to taste. Once the mixture starts to boil remove the pan from the heat.

Finish off by putting in the chicken pieces, baby spinach and creamy milk mixture. Toss, sprinkle with parmesan and serve.

Serves 2

# FRITTATA PACKED WITH ROAST VEGGIES

## Ingredients

4 eggs

2 tbs grated parmesan

1 cup chunky roasted vegetables pieces (include butternut, potatoes, Zucchini, bell peppers, onions)

1/4 cup finely chopped basil leaves

Garden Salad of your choice

## Preparation

Preheat your oven. While waiting, whisk the eggs together and season with salt and pepper.

Heat your chopped vegetables in a non-stick pan for 1 to 2 minutes.

Slowly pour the whisked egg mixture over the heated vegetables and cover. Once the eggs are cooked all the way through liberally sprinkle the basil and parmesan cheese over the top.

Place the pan with all its contents into the preheated oven and allow to grill for 4 minutes. Your frittata should be golden brown.

Slice and serve with a fresh garden salad. Serves 2.

# Beef Kebabs with Teriyaki Sauce and Snow Pea Salad

## Ingredients

22.9 oz (650g) sliced rump steak

2 cups (400g) cooked jasmine rice (Use package instructions)

1thinly sliced Lebanese cucumber

50g mixed lettuce leaves

1/3 cup (80ml) teriyaki sauce

8.8 oz (250g) halved snow peas

## Dressing

1 tsp sesame oil

1 tbs light soy sauce

1-2 tsp wasabi paste (less if you prefer)

1 tsp caster sugar

1 tbs mirin (Japanese rice wine)

1 tbsp rice vinegar

## Preparation

Thread the slices of rump steak onto 8 skewers. Once done place in a dish and pour teriyaki sauce over. Allow to marinate for 10 minutes.

Cook peas in lightly salted water for a minute. Once done, drain and rinse with cold water. Place the peace in a bowl with the lettuce leaves and cucumber slices. Combine all the dressing ingredients and pour over the salad. Toss.

Remove skewers from marinade and allow to cook on a char grilled pan cook for 4 to 5 minutes – approximately 2 minutes per side until cooked.

Served the skewers with the cooked rice and crispy salad. Serves 2.

## Baked Tuna Pasta with Crispy Cheese Topping

### Ingredients

10.6 oz (300g) uncooked macaroni

1.4 oz (40g) butter

2 tbsp plain flour

2 cups low fat milk

3/4 cup low fat grated cheese

15 oz (425g) can flaky tuna (in water – not oil)

### Preparation

Preheat oven to 428°F/392°F (220°C/200°C). Grease a large oven dish.

Cook pasta according to package instructions. Once the pasta is cooked, drain the liquid and make sure you keep1 cup of it. Once the pasta has been rinsed, put it back in the pot that you cooked it in.

Spoon the butter into a medium pan and turn up the heat. Once it has melted add the flour. Keep stirring at all times until the mixture starts bubbling. Now remove from the heat and slowly add the milk. Put the pan back onto the heat and allow to cook for 4 minutes while stirring. The sauce will be thick when it is ready. Now add the grated cheese and season with salt and pepper.

Pour the creamy sauce over the cooked pasta and add the tuna, as well as the remaining liquid from the pasta. Toss.

Place the pasta mixture into the large oven dish and sprinkle cheese over the top. Allow to bake for 10 to 15 minutes, or until the cheese is golden brown and slightly crispy. Serves 4

## CHAR GRILLED SALMON TOPPED WITH TENDER ASPARAGUS

### Ingredients

4 x 6.2 oz (175g) salmon fillets with skin

17.6 oz (500g) baby potatoes chopped in half

8.8 oz (250g) halved and trimmed asparagus

1 small crushed garlic clove

2 tbsp extra virgin olive oil

Olive oil spray

1 tbsp finely chopped flat-leaf parsley

1 tbsp finely shredded tarragon

Juice and zest of half a lime

2 tbsp drained and finely chopped capers

### Preparation

Heat water in a medium sized pot. Add the baby potatoes and a pinch of salt and allow them to cook for 15 minutes or until they are soft.

Coat the salmon with oil using the spray and season to taste. Cook the salmon on either a barbeque or chargrill pan for 3 to 4 minutes a side. The fish should be slightly rare on the inside and crispy on the outside by the time you are done.

Cook asparagus in a pot of boiling salted water for a few minutes until tender. Drain and rinse.  Toss the cooked asparagus with the garlic, parsley and tarragon and lime juice.

Plate the salmon and top with asparagus. Serve with cooked potatoes.  Serves 4.

## TUNA AND SWEET POTATO SALAD ON A BED OF RISONI PASTA

### Ingredients

14.1 oz (400g) sweet potato chopped into chunky pieces

Olive oil cooking spray

7.1 oz (200g) halved baby tomatoes

15 oz (425g) canned tuna

2.6 oz (75g) baby rocket

1 cup dried Risoni pasta

1/4 cup French dressing

### Preparation

Preheat oven to 464ºF/428ºF (240ºC/220ºC). Put the sweet potatoes on a baking tray lined with baking paper, spray with olive oil, and allow to bake for 30 minutes until soft and golden.

Cook pasta according to package instructions. Drain and rinse.

In a medium sized bowl combine the tomato, tuna, rocket, pasta. Drizzle the dressing over and toss before serving. Serve 4

## Lamb With Creamy Kumara

### Ingredients

4 (about 3.5 oz or 100g each) trim lamb leg steaks

26.5 oz (750g) peeled and diced kumara

8.8 oz (250g) cubed zucchini

8.8 oz (250g) cubed yellow squash

1 diced brown onion

8.8 oz (250g) halved cherry tomatoes

1 tsp low fat spread

2 tablespoons heated low-fat milk

2 tsp olive oil

### Preparation

Cook Kumara in the microwave on high for 10 minutes, or until tender. Once done, drain and then season by adding low fat spread, salt and pepper to taste. Mash and add milk if necessary for a smoother consistency.

Heat some of the oil in a pan and then add yellow squash, onion, and zucchini. Cook for about 10 minutes before adding the cherry tomatoes. Continue cooking for 3 more minutes.

Preheat a chargrill or barbeque. Coat the lamb with the leftover oil and season to taste with salt and pepper.  Allow to grill for 6 minutes altogether (3 min per side). Serve lamb with creamy kumara mash and vegetables. Serves 4.

## Spicy Sesame Sirloin Steak with Crispy Cabbage Salad

### Ingredients

3 (about 28.20 oz or 800g) sliced thick sirloin (boneless)

1/4 (about 10.60 oz or 300g) thinly chopped red cabbage, thinly sliced

Steamed rice, to serve

2 tbsp vegetable oil

2 tbsp sesame seeds

2 peeled garlic cloves

3 diced green onions

3 finely sliced red radishes

2 tsp sambal oelek

1/4 cup (60ml) soy sauce

1/4 cup (55g) caster sugar

1/4 cup (60ml) white vinegar

### Preparation

Preheat barbeque. Toast sesame seeds in a small pan by frying them over low heat for only a minute. Pound the sesame seeds

47

and garlic in a mortar with a pestle until ground fine. Combine the soy sauce, sugar, vinegar, oil and sambal oelek and mix with the ground sesame seeds and garlic.

Marinade the strips of sirloin in the sesame mix. Cover with plastic and set aside.

In a medium sized bowl combine green onion, cabbage, radish and half of the dressing. Toss.

Cook beef on heated barbecue for 1 minute a side. Once cooked, drizzle with remaining dressing.

Plate the dish by dividing the cabbage salad amongst 3 bowls and then topping each one with the tender beef. Serve with steamed rice. Serves 3.

## Satay Beef on Crispy Lettuce

### Ingredients

21.20 oz (600g) lean beef mince

4 diced green onions

Steamed jasmine rice

2 tsp peanut oil

8.5 fl oz (250ml) can mild satay sauce

1 peeled and grated carrot

8 large iceberg lettuce leaves

### Preparation

Drizzle some olive oil into a pan. Once heated add the beef mince and fry for 4 minutes. Now add the Satay sauce and continue cooking for 3 minutes.

Add the onion and grated carrot to the dish and allow to cook for a few minutes until carrot has softened. Arrange lettuce onto 4 plates. Top each one with some of the beef

# Beef-Cheek Minestrone on a bed of Risoni Pasta

## Ingredients

17.60 oz (500g) trimmed beef cheeks chopped into cubes

2 tbsp olive oil

4.40 oz (125g) risoni pasta

1 diced onion

Finely diced carrots, garlic cloves and celery stalks (2 each)

1L (4 cups) beef stock

1/2 cup (125ml) red wine

1/3 cup (95g) tomato paste

14.10 oz (400g) can finely diced tomatoes

3.50 oz (100g) baby spinach leaves

Pesto, grissini, pesto and parmesan.

## Preparation

Season beef cubes and then fry in a pan with olive oil in batches for approximately 4 minutes until browned. Stir the cubes around while they cook. Remove the cooked beef and set aside.

Fry the onion, garlic, carrot and celery while stirring for 4 minutes. Now put the beef pack into the pan and add the tomato paste. Cook for 1 minute.

Add stock, season, wine and tomatoes to beef dish. Turn down the heat and bring to a simmer.  Leave to cook for 2 hours. The beef should be tender.

Add the Risoni and cook for 10 more minutes. Finish off by adding the baby spinach leaves. Once they have wilted your dish is ready to be served.

Divide the minestrone into 6 separate bowls and top with some pesto, parmesan shavings and grissini just before serving. Serves 6.

## Chicken Paella

### Ingredients

1 tsp saffron threads

2 tbsp boiling water

1 tbsp olive oil

4 (4.40 oz or 125g each) trimmed and cubed chicken thigh fillets

1 diced red onion

1 1/2 teaspoons smoked sweet paprika

1 medium diced red capsicum

2 cups medium-grain calrose rice

3 cups salt-reduced chicken stock

1 cup thawed frozen peas

1/4 cup finely chopped fresh flat-leaf parsley leaves

1 quartered lemon

### Preparation

Place saffron threads in a bowl of boiling water and allow to stand for 5 minutes.

Heat oil in a heavy duty saucepan. Fry the chicken and onion for 3 to 4 minutes until browned before stirring in the rice, paprika and capsicum.

Pour in the stock and saffron mixture and bring to the boil.

Reduce heat and bring to a simmer. Allow to cook for about 15 minutes and stir every few minutes. Once the rice is soft, add the parsley and peas and season the dish to taste with salt and pepper. Drizzle with lemon and serve. Serves 4.

## SALMON WITH TENDER ASPARAGUS AND BROCCOLINI

### Ingredients

4 x 6.30oz (180g) pieces deboned salmon fillet (with skin on)

1 bunch trimmed, halved broccolini

1 bunch trimmed halved asparagus

1 roughly chopped red onion

2 cloves finely diced garlic cloves

1/2 cup (125ml) peanut oil

1 cup basil leaves

1 tsp sesame oil

1 tsp Chinese five-spice

1/4 cup (80g) hoisin sauce

4cm piece ginger cut into long strips

1.40 oz (40g) baby spinach

Steamed rice to serve.

## Preparation

Slice each salmon fillet into 3 strips. In a medium sized bowl combine the salmon, hoisin sauce, five-spice and 2 tbsp of peanut oil and mix. Season to taste with salt and pepper.

Cook the salmon strips in batches in a frying pan. Heat 1 tsp of peanut oil in the pan for each batch and cook for 1 minutes (30 seconds per side). Set the cooked salmon aside and clean the pan.

Heat leftover peanut oil (about 2 tbsp) over high heat and fry ginger, garlic, onion and stir fry for 2 minutes. Add the asparagus and broccoli and continue frying for a further 3 minutes.

Remove the pan from the stove and stir in sesame oil, basil and spinach. Season to taste. Serve with rice.  Serves 4.

# Hoison Coated Chicken Fillets with Egg Noodles

## Ingredients

21.20 oz (600g) chicken thigh fillets

7.10 oz (200g) dried egg noodles

1/4 cup hoisin sauce

2 tbsp soy sauce

Olive Oil

7.10 oz (200g) trimmed and sliced snow peas

4 diced green onions

2 tbsp Chinese rice wine

2 tsp freshly-grated ginger

## Preparation

In a medium sized bowl combine the soy sauce, ginger, rice wine and hoisin sauce. Pour half the mixture into a separate bowl and add the chicken. Once the chicken is properly coated, cover and place in the fridge for 10 minutes.

Coat a chargrill with olive oil and heat. Cook the chicken for a few minutes on each side and cooked all the way through. Once done, remove and slice into thin slices.

Cook noodles according to package instructions. Add the snow peas to the noodles 30 sec before they are done. Once cooked drain the noodles and snow peas.

In a large serving dish combine the noodle and snow pea mix with the chicken strips and remaining sauce. Serves 4.

# SWEET AND SOUR PORK STIR-FRY

## Ingredients

17.60 oz (500g) pork strips

2 tbsp vegetable oil

Long grain rice (steamed)

3 tsp cornflour

2 bunches trimmed broccolini

Juice from 1 lemon

2 tbsp honey

2 tbsp soy sauce

2 tbsp Chinese rice wine

1 crushed garlic clove

3cm piece grated ginger

## Preparation

In a large bowl mix the ginger, garlic and pork.

Heat some of the olive oil in a large wok. Once heated add half the pork and allow to cook for about 3 minutes or until browned. Place cooked pork in a separate bowl and repeat until all of it is cooked.

Pour the rice wine, honey, 2 tbsp lemon juice and soy sauce into a jug and mix together. Place the cornflour in a little bowl and carefully stir in the liquid mixture until a smooth consistency is formed.

Heat the wok once again and add cooked pork as well as broccolini. Cook for 2 minutes. Now stir in the cornflour and soy mixture and bring to the boil. Stir fry for a further 3 minutes until the broccolini has softened and the sauce has thickened. Serve with steamed rice. Serves 4.

## Egg Noodles Topped with Ginger and Soy Pork

### Ingredients

4 (5.3 oz or 150g each) lean pork butterfly steaks

15.90 oz (450g) Egg noodles

2 tsp sesame seeds

5cm piece peeled and diced ginger

Canola Oil

1/4 cup oyster sauce

1 bunch diced and trimmed choy sum

2 cloves crushed garlic

1/4 cup soy sauce

2 tsp black pepper

### Preparation

Cook noodles according to package instructions.

Mix the soy sauce, garlic, black pepper and ginger in a medium sized bowl. Add the pork steaks and coat thoroughly.

Heat some oil in a large frying pan and proceed to cook each pork steak for about 3 minutes per side. Keep the remaining marinade to use later.

Coat a large wok with some oil and heat. Once heated toast sesame seeds for a minute until golden brown. Now pour in the remaining marinade and the choy sum. Cook for a few minutes to allow the choy sum to wilt.

Remove the pork mixture from the wok and add the cooked noodles, 2 tbsp of cold water and oyster sauce.  Cook for a further 2 minutes until the noodle dish is heated all the way through. Serve with pork dish. Serves 4.

## Snapper with a Side of Sweetcorn Salsa

### Ingredients

4 (5.30 oz 150g each) halved snapper fish fillets

1/2 finely shredded small red onion

1 finely chopped red capsicum

1 long green chili, sliced into long pieces

2 tbsp ground coriander leaves

2 (17.60 oz or 500g) trimmed corn cobs, trimmed

14.10 oz (400g) can chickpeas (Drain fluid and rinse)

1 large diced avocado

1/4 cup lime juice

1/4 cup olive oil

Fresh coriander leaves

### Preparation

Cook corn in the microwave on high for 5 minutes. Once cooked remove and place in a bowl of ice water.

In a large bowl combine the avocado, capsicum, onion, chili, chickpeas, and diced coriander. Remove the corn from the ice water and remove all the kernels. Add the kernels to the avocado mixture.

Combine 2 tbsp of olive oil with 2 tablespoons lime juice and season with salt and pepper. Pour this over the avocado mixture and toss.

Heat oil in a nonstick frying pan. Cooked seasoned fish for 2 minutes on each side until cooked all the way through.

Divide the fish amongst 4 serving plates and drizzle with leftover lime juice. Top with fresh coriander and salsa before serving. Serves 4.

# TENDER PORK WITH A PINEAPPLE SALSA AND SNOW PEAS

## Ingredients

4 (about 4.40 oz or 125g each) pork loin steaks

250g trimmed and halved snow peas

Olive oil

2 halved and thinly sliced cucumbers

## Pineapple salsa

2 tbsp chopped fresh coriander

1 tsp fish sauce

1 tbsp fresh lime juice

1/2 (19.40 oz or 500g) peeled and cored pineapple cut into 5mm slices

1 long fresh red chili – remove seeds and chop finely

## Preparation

For a delicious pineapple salsa combine the coriander, chili, pineapple, fish sauce and lime juice and mix together.

Heat a barbeque grill. Thoroughly coat each piece of pork with olive oil and then place on the heated grill. Allow to cook for 4 minutes per side or longer if you prefer. Once the pork is cooked remove it and set it aside to rest for a few minutes

Cook the snow peas in a pot of boiling water for 3 minutes. Once cooked, drain and rinse with cold water. Transfer the snow peas into a bowl and add the cucumber. Toss.

Divide the snow pea and cucumber mixture among 4 plates. Top with cucumber salsa and grilled pork. Serves 4.

## Hearty Italian Pork and Broccoli Soup

### Ingredients

17.60 oz (500g) Large Italian pork sausages

7.10 oz (200g) medium sized broccoli florets

1.80 oz (50g) dried pasta of your choice

1 diced brown onion

1 diced red capsicum

2 diced celery stalks

1 1/2 cups chicken stock

15.20 oz (430g) can thick tomato soup

### Preparation

Remove the meat from the pork sausage casings and roll into small meatballs.

Cook the meatballs in a nonstick pan for a few minutes until browned. Remove the cooked meatballs and set aside. Now add the celery and diced onion and cook for 4 minutes while stirring.

Add the stock, soup, meatballs, capsicum, and 1/2 cup cold water and bring to the boil. Reduce heat and bring to a simmer. Allow to cook for a further 8 minutes until meatballs and properly cooked.

Add the pasta and broccoli and simmer for 4 more minutes or until the pasta is cooked. Serves 4.

## Juicy Lamb Sosaties (Kebabs)

### Ingredients

21.20 oz (600g) lamb leg steaks

24.70 oz (700g) peeled and cubed orange sweet potato

2 tbsp olive oil

1 lemon, rind finely grated, juiced

Oz (70g) rocket leaves

Lemon wedges

1 tablespoon honey

2 crushed cloves of garlic

12 rosemary sprigs

### Preparation

Remove leaves from rosemary sprigs, reserving 2 tablespoons leaves. Soak rosemary skewers in cold water for 30 minutes. Drain. Chop reserved leaves.

Cut lamb into 2cm cubes. Thread onto rosemary skewers. Place in a ceramic dish. Whisk rind, honey, garlic, reserved rosemary, 1 tablespoon oil and 1 tablespoon lemon juice in a jug. Pour over kebabs. Turn to coat. Cover and refrigerate for 30 minutes.

Place sweet potato onto a microwave-safe plate. Cover. Microwave on HIGH (100%) for 6 to 8 minutes or until just tender. Drain. Drizzle with remaining oil. Season with salt and pepper.

Preheat barbecue plate on high heat. Reduce to medium. Lightly grease. Cook sweet potato for 2 minutes each side or until golden. Transfer to a plate. Cover with foil. Add kebabs to barbecue and cook for 2 minutes each side for medium or until cooked to your liking.

Place sweet potato onto serving plates. Top with lamb kebabs and serve with rocket and lemon wedges.

## Roast Lamb and Veggies

### Ingredients

6 cutlet racks of lamb (x2)

2 tbsp olive oil

21.20 oz (600g) halved baby potatoes

5 medium sized carrots

4 quartered medium sized red onions

5.30 oz (150g) baby spinach leaves

Salt

Freshly ground black pepper

### Preparation

Preheat oven to 428°F (220°C). Place the onions and potatoes on a roasting tray lined with baking paper and season with salt and pepper. Place the tray in the oven and bake for 25 minutes.

Season the racks of lamb with salt and pepper. Drizzle some olive into a large pan and heat. Fry the seasoned racks of lamb for about 3 minutes per side until they have browned.

Now remove the pan from the heat and arrange the baby carrots around the lamb. Place the pan in the oven and allow to cook for a further 20 minutes. The Lamb should be cooked all the way through and the vegetable should be tender. Now place the cooked lamb on a plate and cover with foil. Set aside to rest for a few minutes.

Steam baby spinach leaves until they have wilted. Serve carved lamb with roasted vegetables and spinach leaves. Serves 4.

Steam or microwave spinach. Carve the lamb. Serve with the roasted vegetables and spinach. Serves 4.

## Lamb filled Shepherd's Pie with Crispy Cheese Topping

### Ingredients

17.60 oz (500g) lamb mince

30 oz (850g) peeled and cubed potatoes

1 tbsp olive oil

1/2 cup (125g) tomato paste

1/2 cup (125ml) milk

1.10 oz (30g) butter

2 tbsp plain flour

1 finely diced medium sized onion

1 peeled and diced carrot

2 finely diced zucchini

2 cups (500ml) beef stock

1 1/2 tbsp Worcestershire sauce

1 1/3 cups (115g) grated cheddar cheese

2 dried bay leaves

## Preparation

Heat some olive oil in a large pan. Once heated add the diced onion and carrot and fry for a minute while stirring. Now increase the heat and add the mince. Cook for about 5 minutes, or until the mince has browned. Add the flour and zucchini and cook for another minute.

Now add the tomato paste, stock, Worcestershire sauce and bay leaves to the mince. Turn down the heat and allow to simmer for 15 minutes until the sauce has thickened.

Boil some water in a small pot and then add the potatoes. Cook for around 10 minutes, or until potatoes are tender. Drain and mash until silky smooth. Stir in butter and milk and season with salt and pepper to taste.

Preheat grill. Place the cooked mincemeat into a large oven proof dish. Top with the creamy mash and grated cheddar. Place under the grill for 4 minutes, or until cheese is brown and slightly crispy. Serves 4.

## TRADITIONAL SPAGHETTI BOLOGNAISE

### Ingredients

14.10 oz (400g) lean beef mince

1 tbsp olive oil

26 oz (737g) tomato paste with basil

1 finely chopped onion

21.20 oz (600g) Spaghetti

14.10 oz (400g) can brown rinsed lentils

1finely chopped celery stick

1 large grated zucchini

1 large diced carrot

Grated parmesan cheese

### Preparation

Heat some oil in a large pan and add the zucchini, carrot, onion and celery. Cook for 3 to 4 minutes until onion has browned slightly. Now add the mince and continue cooking while stirring for a further 6 minutes, or until mince has browned.

Add lentils and pasta sauce to browned mince and reduce heat. Simmer for 15 minutes until the sauce has thickened. Season to taste with salt and pepper.

Cook spaghetti according to package instructions until al Dente. Drain. Serve spaghetti with parmesan cheese. Serves 6.

Meanwhile, cook pasta in a saucepan of boiling water, following packet directions, until tender. Drain. Divide pasta between bowls. Spoon over sauce. Serve with cheese. Serves 4.

## Spicy grilled Fish and Fresh Vegetables

### Ingredients

4 (5.30 oz or 150g each) firm white fish fillets

2 tbsp olive oil

1 tsp smoked paprika

1 1/3 cups flat-leaf parsley leaves

Juice from 1/2 lemon

2 thinly diced zucchini

2 baby eggplants, sliced diagonally

1 halved and chopped red capsicum

oz (150g) diced button mushrooms

Crispy wholewheat bread

### Preparation

Drizzle some olive oil into a large pan and heat on medium high heat. While you wait, season the fish with oil and paprika. Place the zucchini, capsicum, mushrooms and eggplant in bowl and coat with 1 tbsp of oil. Season the vegetables to taste with salt and pepper.

Cook the vegetables on a heated barbeque plate for 8 to 10 minutes whilst turning. Once they have browned, place them in a bowl and toss with parsley and 1 1/2 tbsp of lemon juice.

Cook the seasoned fish on the same grill for 2 minutes per side and then serve with wholewheat bread and golden brown vegetables. Serves 4.

# Chicken and Crunchy Broccoli Stir-Fry

## Ingredients

14.10 oz (400g) sliced chicken breast fillets

Olive oil spray

1thinly sliced red onion

14.10 oz (400g) peeled and cubed pumpkin

10.60 oz (300g) broccoli florets

2 garlic cloves (crushed)

2 tbsp dry sherry

2 tsp caster sugar

1 tbsp reduced salt soy sauce

1/3 cup (80ml) water

2 tsp Sambal Oelek

Steamed rice

## Preparation

Drizzle some olive oil into a large wok and heat. Once heated add the chicken and allow to cook for a few minutes until it has browned.

In a small bowl combine the sugar, sherry and soy sauce and stir until the sugar has dissolved.

Drizzle more olive oil into the wok and heat. Add the onion, garlic and Sambal Oelek and stir fry for a few minutes. Now add the water and cubed pumpkin. Continue cooking for a few minutes until the pumpkin has softened. Add the broccoli florets and cook for a further 3 minutes.

Add the browned chicken and soy sauce mixture to the vegetable mix and combine. Heat for 2 minutes before serving. Serves 4.

## KUMARA AND DRIED TOMATO MASH WITH VEAL STEAKS

### Ingredients

4 (3.50 oz or 100g each) thin veal steaks

1 1/2 tbsp olive oil

1 chopped garlic clove

1/4 cup chopped semi-dried tomatoes

28.20 oz (800g) peeled and cubed Kumara

Steamed green beans (to serve)

1/4 cup warm low fat milk

1/4 cup balsamic vinegar

### Preparation

Fill a saucepan with water and bring to the boil. Add the kumara cubes and allow to cook for around 10 minutes. Once cooked, place the kumara in a medium sized bowl and mash. Add the milk and sun-dried tomatoes to the mash and season with salt and pepper.

Heat olive oil in a large frying pan and fry the veal steaks for 2 minutes per side. In a small bowl combine the garlic and balsamic vinegar.

Serve veal steaks with Kumara mash and green beans and drizzle the balsamic vinegar over the dish. Serves 4.

## KUMARA AND CAPSICUM FRITTATA

### Ingredients

1chopped red capsicum

1 medium 14.10 oz (400g) peeled and cubed orange Kumara

6 eggs

2 tbsp olive oil

2 finely chopped garlic cloves

1/3 cup grated parmesan cheese

### Preparation

Preheat oven to 356°F (180°C)

Fill a medium sized pot with water and bring to the boil. Add the sweet potato and cook for a few minutes until soft. Remove from the water and drain.

Heat olive oil in a pan and fry the garlic and capsicum for a few minutes, stirring all the time. In a small bowl beat the eggs and season them with salt and pepper. Pour the eggs into a greased 18cm x 28 cm slice pan. Top with the fried garlic and capsicum and tender sweet potatoes and finish off by sprinkling with parmesan.

Place into the oven and cook for 20 minutes. Remove and allow to cool before slicing and serving. Serves 8.

## Broccoli and Snow Pea Fritters with Yoghurt

### Ingredients

1 cup (130g) plain flour

2 peeled and crushed cloves of garlic

3/4 cup (180ml) water

Canola or Sunflower Oil

1/2 cup plain yoghurt

10.60 oz (300g) broccoli florets

3,5 oz (100g) snow peas

Salt & freshly ground pepper

Steamed rice, to serve

### Preparation

In a medium sized bowl combine the broccoli and snow peas with the flour, water, and half the garlic and mix. Season to taste with salt and pepper.

Fill a wok to one-third with sunflower or canola oil and heat. Once the oil is hot, spoon heaped tablespoons of batter in and fry for 5 minutes. Turn the fritters from time to time while they are frying.

Once cooked, remove from the oil and drain. Keep doing this until all the batter has been used.

Combine the plain yoghurt with the leftover garlic and serve with steamed rice and crunchy fritters. Serves 4.

## Walnut and Cranberry Zucchini Bread

### Ingredients

3 large grated zucchinis

3/4 cup (75g) chopped and toasted walnuts

1/3 cup dried cranberries

1 1/3 cups (295g) caster sugar

2 tsp vanilla extract

1/2 cup (100g) brown sugar

3 beaten eggs

1 tsp ground cinnamon

2 2/3 cups (400g) plain flour

1 tsp bicarbonate of soda

1/2 tsp baking powder

1/4 tsp mixed spice

6.80 fl oz (200ml) sunflower oil

Brie Cheese (to serve)

### Preparation

Preheat oven to 302°F (150°C).

Sift the flour, baking powder, bicarbonate of soda and spices into a mixing bowl. Now add the beaten eggs, vanilla, nuts, zucchini, cranberries, caster sugar, brown sugar and salt and mix together.

Once the mixture is properly combined transfer it into a greased 2L loaf pan.

Put the loaf pan into the oven and bake for about 1 hour, or slightly longer if necessary.

Once done, remove the loaf from the oven and allow to cool. Serve with slices of Brie Cheese.

## PORK STIR-FRY WITH PICKLED LEBANESE CUCUMBERS

**Ingredients**

17.60 oz (500g) lean pork mince

1 Lebanese cucumber

3 thinly sliced spring onions

3.50 oz (100g) snow peas

1 long finely diced red chili (remove seeds)

1/3 cup coriander leaves

2 tbsp each soy and oyster sauce

1 tbsp sweet chili sauce

1 tbsp cornflour

2 tsp caster sugar

2 tbsp rice vinegar

2 tsp grated fresh ginger

5.60 oz (160g) rice noodles

**Preparation**

Peel the cucumber and then cut it down the middle before removing the seeds. Using a peeler, cut the cucumber halves into long strips. In a small bowl combine the chili, sugar and 1 tbsp of vinegar and stir. In a separate bowl combine the cucumber strips with the vinegar mixture. Cover and allow for stand for a few minutes.

Pour half a cup of water into a bowl and then add the soy, oyster and sweet chili sauce. Stir to combine. In a separate bowl combine 1 tbsp of vinegar with the cornflour.

Heat oil in a wok. Once heated add the spring onion and ginger and stir fry for a minute. Now add the pork mince and cook for a few minutes. Once the meat has browned, pour in the sauce mixture and coriander leaves and continue cooking for 2 minutes. Now add the snow peas and stir fry for another minute.

Serve the cooked pork with rice noodles and a side of pickled cucumber. Serves 4.

# Scrumptious Lunches

### Delicious Chicken Tortilla

**Ingredients**

1 sliced chicken breast

1 tsp olive oil

1 finely chopped onion

1roughly chopped red or green pepper

A few small tortillas

1 peeled and grated carrot

1 cup of lettuce

14 oz. drained kidney beans

1 tbsp crème fraiche

Salt and pepper

**Preparation**

Fry the onion and pepper in the tsp of olive oil for approximately 2 minutes.

Add the chicken pieces and continue frying until the chicken is cooked and nicely browned.

In a separate bowl combine and crème fraiche and kidney beans and mash.

Spread the mixture onto a few tortillas and then add the chicken, lettuce leaves and carrots before you roll it up. Guaranteed to be delicious!

## Thai Chicken Noodle Salad

### Ingredients

2 chopped chicken breasts

2 chopped cloves of garlic

1 lime (use juice and zest)

1 tsp oil

2 tbsp chopped coriander

1 orange (use juice and zest)

¼ cucumber sliced

½ chopped red chili

3 oz. halved blanched beans

1 cup cooked noodles

3 sliced spring onions

I tsp honey

### Preparation

Place the chicken in a medium sized dish and cover with the juice and zest from the lime. Place in the refrigerator and leave to marinate for approximately 30 min.

Place the tsp of olive oil in a frying pan and fry the garlic and chicken until the chicken is properly cooked (should take about 8 min).

In a large bowl combine the onion, coriander, beans, cucumber, noodles and chili.

Make a dressing out of the honey and orange and drizzle over salad

To serve, place salad in plates and finish off by placing the fried chicken on top.

# Sweet and Sour Chicken Salad

## Ingredients

4 large chicken breasts (boneless and skinless)

Teriyaki sauce (enough to marinate chicken in)

8 won tons

1 head lettuce chopped

2 tbsp + 2 tsp vinegar

3 tbsp + 2 tsp canola oil

¾ tsp paprika

Ground black pepper

1 tbsp sweet and sour sauce

1 tbsp sesame seeds (toasted)

1 tsp salt

¼ cup green onions

## Preparation

Marinate chicken pieces in Teriyaki sauce for a few hours before baking or placing in microwave until cooked through. Cut into cubes.

Fry won ton in 1 tbsp canola oil and drain.

Combine the vinegar, remaining canola oil, paprika, black pepper, sweet and sour sauce and salt in a pot and bring to a boil. Once boiling starts turn off heat and allow to cool.

In a salad bowl combine the lettuce, chicken, sesame seeds, and green onions.

Just before serving add the dressing and won tons and your sticky delicious salad is ready!

## Corn, Avo and Brown Rice Salad

### Ingredients

3 cups cooked brown rice

½ cup toasted almonds

1 avocado

2 ears of cooked corn

1 tsp lemon juice

1 tsp canola oil

1 tsp brown rice vinegar

1 tsp tamari soy sauce

4 chopped large lettuce leaves

### Preparation

Cook rice according to package instructions

Peel the avo and pit before mashing with the cooked rice.

Remove the corn from the cob and add to the mixture. Also add the onions and almonds.

In a small bowl combine the oil, vinegar, lemon juice, and tamari sauce. Mix together and pour all over salad. Serve chilled.

# TURKEY AND COLESLAW SANDWICH

## Ingredients

2 cups grated carrot and cabbage (mixed)

2 tbsp low fat Italian salad dressing

2 slices of rye bread

9 oz. thinly slices turkey breast (cooked)

3 slices provolone cheese

1 thinly sliced tomato

Cucumber slices

## Preparation

Place coleslaw mix in a bowl and combine with Italian dressing.

Place rye bread slices on a plate and top with turkey, cheese slices, tomato slices, coleslaw, and cucumber slices.

Close sandwich and toast in a heated pan – 4 min per side or until cheese is melted.

## Vegetarian Open Sandwich

**Ingredients**

2 tsp Dijon mustard

1/4 cup grated carrot

1/2 cup broccoli florets (small)

2 toasted whole-wheat English Muffins

1/4 cup roughly chopped red bell pepper

1/2 cup shredded Monterey Jack Cheese (Low Fat)

**Preparation**

Turn on oven (grill)

Spread Dijon mustard over all sides of English muffin and top with broccoli, carrots and bell peppers. Finish of with shredded cheese.

Place under grill for a few min, or until cheese has melted.

# Five-spice Salmon with Broccolini and Asparagus

## Ingredients

4 x 6.3 oz (180g) pieces salmon fillet, pin-boned, skin on

1 tsp Chinese five-spice

1/4 cup (80g) hoisin sauce

1/2 cup (125ml) peanut oil

2 cloves garlic, thinly sliced

4cm piece ginger, cut into julienne (matchsticks)

1 red onion, thickly sliced

1 bunch broccolini, trimmed, halved widthwise

1 bunch asparagus, trimmed, halved widthwise

1.4 oz (40g) baby spinach

1 cup basil leaves

1 tsp sesame oil

Steamed rice (optional), to serve

## Preparation

Using a sharp knife, cut each piece of fish into 3 lengthwise. Place in a large bowl. Add five-spice, hoisin sauce and 2 tbs peanut oil. Season with salt and pepper. Gently toss to combine.

Heat 1 tbs peanut oil in a large frying pan over high heat. Add half the fish and cook for 30 seconds each side for medium-rare or until cooked to your liking. Transfer to a plate. Repeat with another 1 tbs peanut oil and remaining fish. Wipe pan clean.

Heat remaining 2 tbs peanut oil in pan over high heat. Add garlic, ginger and onion, and stir-fry for 2 minutes or until onion is soft. Add broccolini and asparagus, and stir-fry for a further 3 minutes or until vegetables are tender. Remove from heat and stir in spinach, basil and sesame oil, then season.

Divide the vegetables and fish among plates. Serve with rice, if using. Serves 5

# Roasted Pumpkin and Spinach Salad with a Walnut Dressing

## Ingredients

5.3 oz (150g) baby spinach leaves

¼ cup olive oil

31.75 oz (900g) peeled and cubed butternut

## Dressing

1 1/2 tbsp lemon juice

1 crushed garlic clove

1 tbsp extra-virgin olive oil

100g (1 cup) roughly diced walnuts

## Preparation

Preheat oven to 446°F (230°C). Scatter the pumpkin cubes onto a lined baking tray and drizzle with olive oil. Place the tray into the oven and bake for 20 minutes, or until the pumpkin is tender.

For the dressing, heat some oil in a non-stick frying pan. Add the walnuts and fry for about 5 minutes, or until they are toasted and crisp. Remove the pan from the heat and carefully stir in the lemon juice and garlic. Season to taste with salt and pepper.

Arrange the spinach leaves onto a serving plate. Top with tender pumpkin and drizzle with walnut dressing. Serves 8.

# Barbequed Snapper and Tender Vegetables

## Ingredients

4 deboned snapper fillets (don't remove skin)

3 chopped zucchinis

2.8 oz (80g) pitted kalamata olives

1 halved red capsicum (remove seeds)

1/3 cup (80ml) olive oil

2 tbsp red wine vinegar

1 quartered red onion

2 sliced Japanese eggplants

3 roma tomatoes, halved

8 thyme sprigs

1/4 bunch basil

## Preparation

Preheat a barbeque to medium high heat. In a large bowl combine the capsicum, eggplant, tomatoes and zucchini. Drizzle the vegetables with 2 tbsp of olive oil and add the thyme from 4 of the sprigs. Season with sufficient salt and pepper and toss to combine.

Remove the capsicum halves from the bowl and place them on the heated grill to cook for 2 minutes a side. They should be slightly browned on each side. Remove the capsicum and then place the rest of the vegetables on the grill and cook for 3 minutes. Turn the vegetables while they are on the grill to cook on all sides. Now remove the vegetables and place them all back in the same bowl.

Place the deboned snapper fillets on a large tray. Drizzle with olive oil and scatter the remaining thyme over. Place the fillets on the grill and allow to cook for 2 minutes per side. Once done, set the snapper aside for a few minutes before serving.

To finish off the vegetable dish, stir in the kalamata olives and drizzle leftover olive oil and vinegar over the dish. Sprinkle some basil over and then toss to combine.

Serve tender vegetables with grilled snapper. Serves 4.

## Roast Beef, Spinach and Caramelized Onions on Toasted Rye

### Ingredients

7.10 oz (200g) roast beef shavings

2 red onions sliced into thin strips

8 slices rye bread

5.30 oz (150g) grated cheese

1 tbsp balsamic vinegar

1.80 oz (50g) baby spinach leaves

1 tbsp olive oil

1 tbsp brown sugar

### Preparation

Heat some olive oil in a pan. Once heated add onion slices and allow to cook, while stirring, for about 10 minutes. Now add the brown sugar and vinegar and allow to cook for a few more minutes until the onions have caramelized.

Preheat a grill. Once heated toast the rye bread on one side for 2 minutes. Turn the bread around and top with grated cheese. Grill for a few more minutes until the cheese has melted. Remove from the grill and top with roast beef, spinach and onions. Serves 4.

## JUICY LAMB WRAPS

### Ingredients

Olive Oil

17.60 oz (500g) lamb rump steak

2 x 2.50 oz (70g) baby lettuce leaves and beetroot salad mix.

4 Spinach and Herb Wraps

1.20 oz (35g) pkt taco seasoning

### Preparation

Remove the fat from the rump steaks and slice each one into thin strips. Place the strips in a bowl and season with taco seasoning.

Heat some olive oil in a frying pan. Cook the lamb strips in batches until all of it is cooked through. 2 minutes per batch should suffice and keep lamb tender.

Divide the salad mixture amongst 4 spinach and herb wraps and then top each one with 1/4 of the cooked lamb. Roll each wrap to enclose filling before serving. Serves 4.

# Baguette Topped with Roast Beef, Mustard, and Salad

## Ingredients

1/4 cup wholegrain mustard

2 chopped up medium tomatoes

2 tbsp sliced black olives

2 x 22cm halved wholewheat baguettes

8 slices (8.80 oz or 250g) rare roast beef

2 tbsp sliced pickled jalapeno chilies

1/2 thinly sliced green capsicum, thinly sliced

2 diced iceberg lettuce leaves

3 slices cheese (halved)

1 small peeled and grated carrot

1 Lebanese cucumber cut into thin strips

## Preparation

Spread mustard over each baguette half and then top two of the halves with beef, carrot, capsicum, lettuce, tomato, cucumber, chilies and cheese. Close each sandwich it's other half before serving. Serves 4.

# Something Sweet - A Delectable Selection

## Fluffy Carrot and Date Dessert

### Ingredients

1/2 cup self-raising flour

1 tsp vanilla essence

1/2 small grated carrot

1/2 tsp bicarbonate of soda

1 tbsp brown sugar

1/2 cup (125g) finely chopped and pitted fresh dates

1 egg

1.1 oz (30g) low-fat dairy spread

1 tsp pure icing sugar

Whipped cream, to serve

## Preparation

Preheat your oven to 374°F (190°C). Grease and line 4 medium sized ramekins.

Pour 1/2 cup of water and the dates into a pot and bring to the boil. Lower the heat and simmer for 2 minutes before stirring in the bicarbonate of soda.

In a medium sized bowl combine the dairy spread and sugar and beat with an electric mixer. Now add the egg and vanilla essence and continue mixing. Once properly combined, stir in the carrot and date mixture. Sift the flour over the date mixture and combine.

Divide the mixture among the ramekins and place them in a baking tray. Place into the heated oven and allow to bake for 20 minutes. Once done, remove the baking tray and allow to cool for 5 minutes. Transfer onto a serving plate and dust with icing sugar. Serve with fresh whipped cream.

## Refreshing Vanilla Yoghurt and Mango Pops

**Ingredients**

3 chopped up ripe mangoes

260g (1 cup) low fat vanilla yoghurt

**Preparation**

Place the mangoes into a food processor and blend until smooth. Remove the mango puree and combine with the vanilla yoghurt in a separate bowl.

Transfer the vanilla and mango mixture into an ice tray that has at least 8 80 ml sections.

Place the tray in the freezer and leave to freeze for at least 8 hours. Refreshing and delicious!

## Pecan, Almond and Dried Fruit Bars

### Ingredients

45g (1/3 cup) roughly chopped pecan nuts

60g (1/3 cup) chopped blanched almonds

25g (1/3 cup) diced dried apples

70g (1/3 cup) diced dried apricots

90g (1 cup) rolled oats

1 tbsp light olive oil

2 tbsp maple syrup

### Preparation

Preheat oven to 180°C. In a medium bowl combine the rolled oats with the olive oil and maple syrup.

Scatter the oats onto a baking tray and bake in the preheated oven for 5 minutes. Remove from the oven and scatter the almonds and pecans over the oat mixture.

Stir to combine and then place back into the oven for 6 more minutes. The nuts should be brown and crispy once they are done.

Remove the oat mixture from the oven and transfer the contents into a large bowl. Now add the dried fruit and mix.

Store the bars in an airtight container. Sprinkle the bars over tinned fruit, yoghurt, or cereal.

## Walnut and Orange Loaf

### Ingredients

1 cup diced walnuts

2.10 oz (60g) melted butter

1 cup orange juice

1 whisked egg

2 cups self-raising flour

1 tsp bicarbonate of soda

1cup (185g) diced dried apricots

1 cup caster sugar

### Preparation

Preheat oven to 338°F (170°C). Grease a 6cm deep, 12cm x 20cm (base) loaf pan and then line it with baking paper.

Pour 1 cup of cold water into a pot and bring to the boil. Now turn down the heat and add the apricots. Allow to simmer for 5 minutes until apricots are tender. Remove the apricots and keep 100 ml of the liquid used to boil them.

Sift the flour into a medium sized bowl and then add the bicarbonate of soda, sugar and walnuts and mix together.

In a separate bowl combine the orange juice, egg, butter and liquid that you reserved from the apricots and blend. Combine this wet mixture with the dry mixture and mix thoroughly.

Spoon this batter into the greased pan and put it in the oven to bake for 50 minutes. Once done, remove and allow to cool for 10 minutes. Serves 10.

## Mixed Berry and Banana Smoothie

### Ingredients

1/2 cup low-fat milk

1/2 cup low-fat vanilla yoghurt

4 ice cubes

1 large sliced banana

2 tsp honey

1/2 cup mixed berries

2 teaspoons wheat germ

### Preparation

Place all the ingredients in a blender and blend until smooth.

Serves 2.

## Banana Bread at its Best

### Ingredients

1/2 cup melted butter (for greasing)

1/2 cup (125ml) skim milk

2/3 cup (140g) brown sugar

2 beaten eggs

2 mashed bananas (overripe)

1.8 oz (50g) butter

1 tsp ground cinnamon

1 3/4 cups (265g) self-raising flour

1/4 cup (40g) plain flour

### Preparation

Preheat oven to 356°F (180°C). Using the melted butter, grease an 11 x 21 cm loaf pan and then line it with baking paper.

Sift plain and self-raising flour into a bowl. Add the sugar. In a separate bowl combine the eggs, milk, butter, and mashed banana and stir. Combine the wet and dry ingredients and mix thoroughly.

Spoon the smooth batter into the greased loaf pan and then place in the oven to bake for 45 minutes. Once done, remove the loaf and set it aside to cool for at least 5 minutes before removing and serving. Serves 10.

## Vanilla, Banana and Honey Smoothie

### Ingredients

1/4 cup milk

1 1/2 tbsp honey

1 large sliced banana

4 ice cubes

3/4 cup creamy low fat vanilla yoghurt

### Preparation

Place all the ingredients into a blender and blend until smooth and frothy. Serves 1.

## Strawberry Banana Yoghurt Muffins

### Ingredients

1 cup strawberry yoghurt

2 mashed bananas

1/2 cup caster sugar

1 egg

2/3 cup vegetable oil

1 3/4 cups self-raising flour

### Preparation

Preheat oven to 356°F (180°C). Grease a muffin pan. The pan must be big enough for 12 muffins.

Sift the flour and sugar into a large mixing bowl. In a separate bowl combine the egg, yoghurt, oil and 1 cup of mashed banana. Slowly combine the flour and yoghurt mixture and stir gently until the batter is properly combined.

Using a large spoon, transfer the batter into the muffin pan. Place the pan in the preheated oven and allow to bake for around 25 minutes. Once done, remove the muffins and allow them to cool slightly before removing them from the pan.

## Light and Fluffy Lemon Pudding

### Ingredients

1 cup (150g) self-raising flour

1 cup (215g) caster sugar

3 tbsp icing sugar

2 tbsp melted butter

1 1/3 cups (330ml) low fat milk

4 eggs (separate white and yolk)

2/3 cup (160ml) fresh lemon juice

1 tbsp grated lemon rind

Sweetened whipped cream, to serve

### Preparation

Preheat oven to 356°F (180ºC). Using the butter, grease 6 250 ml (1 cup) capacity ramekins

In a medium sized mixing bowl combine the flour, milk, egg yolks, lemon rind, lemon juice, 2/3cup (140g) caster sugar and mix until creamy.

Beat egg whites in a separate bowl using an electric mixer until light and fluffy. Slowly beat in the rest of the caster sugar - the egg white should thicken somewhat.

Slowly fold the fluffy egg white mix into the creamy lemon mixture before dividing the batter among the ramekins. Place the ramekins in a large roasting pan and then fill the pan with water. The water should come halfway up the ramekins.

Bake the lemon dessert for 35 minutes. Once done, remove the ramekins and dust each one with icing sugar. Serve with fresh whipped cream. Serves 6.

## Berry Delight Smoothie

### Ingredients

1/3 cup milk

1 tablespoon maple syrup

2/3 cup low fat vanilla yoghurt

4 ice cubes

5.30 oz (150g) diced strawberries

1/2 cup raspberries

### Preparation

Place all the ingredients in a blender and blend until creamy and frothy. Serves 2

# BIBLIOGRAPHY

Murkoff H, Eisenberg A and Hathaway S 1984. What to Expect when You're Expecting.

Simon and Schuster: Kingsway, London. The Baby Blues

Pregnancy and Childbirth: Overcome your Fears and Convert it into Joy.

Pregnancy Guide: Guide to Preparing for Parenthood

Encyclopedia of Natural Medicine Revised 2nd Edition: Michael Murray N.D. and Joseph Pizzorno N.D.

Alternative Medicine: The Definitive Guide; Second Edition: Larry Trivieri, JR Editor, Introduced by Burton Goldberg.

Alternative Cures: Bill Gottlieb

# MORE BOOKS BY JOHN MCARTHUR

## Hypothyroidism

**Hypothyroidism: The Hypothyroidism Solution.** Hypothyroidism Natural Treatment and Hypothyroidism Diet for Under Active Or Slow Thyroid, Causing Weight Loss Problems, Fatigue, Cardiovascular Disease. John McArthur (Author), Cheri Merz (Editor)

## Fibromyalgia And Chronic Fatigue

**Fibromyalgia And Chronic Fatigue:** A Step-By-Step Guide For Fibromyalgia Treatment And Chronic Fatigue Syndrome Treatment. Includes Fibromyalgia Diet And Chronic Fatigue Diet And Lifestyle Guidelines. John McArthur (Author), Cheri Merz (Editor)

## Yeast Infection

**Candida Albicans:** Yeast Infection Treatment. Treat Yeast Infections With This Home Remedy. The Yeast Infection Cure. John McArthur (Author)

## Heart Disease

**Hypertension - High Blood Pressure:** How To Lower Blood Pressure Permanently In 8 Weeks Or Less, The Hypertension Treatment,

Diet and Solution. John McArthur (Author)

**Cholesterol Myth:** Lower Cholesterol Won't Stop Heart Disease. Healthy Cholesterol Will. Cholesterol Recipe Book & Cholesterol Diet. Lower Cholesterol Naturally Keep Cholesterol Healthy. John McArthur (Author), Cheri Merz (Editor)

**Heart Disease Prevention and Reversal:** How To Prevent, Cure and Reverse Heart Disease Naturally For A Healthy Heart. John McArthur (Author)

## Diabetes

**Diabetes Diet:** Diabetes Management Options. Includes a Diabetes Diet Plan with Diabetic Meals and Natural Diabetes Food, Herbs and Supplements for Total Diabetes Control. Delicious Recipes. John McArthur (Author), Corinne Watson (Editor)

**Diabetes Cooking:** 93 Diabetes Recipes for Breakfast, Lunch, Dinner, Snacks and Smoothies. A Guide to Diabetes Foods to Help You Prepare Healthy Delicious ... Diabetic Meals and Natural Diabetes Food) John McArthur (Author), Corinne Watson (Editor)

## Stress and Anxiety

**From Stressful to Successful in 4 Easy Steps:** Stress at Work? Stress in Relationship? Be Stress Free. End Stress and Anxiety. Excellent

Stress Management, Stress Control and Stress Relief Techniques. John McArthur (Author)

**Anxiety and Panic Attacks:** Anxiety Management. Anxiety Relief. The Natural And Drug Free Relief For Anxiety Attacks, Panic Attacks And Panic Disorder. John McArthur (Author), Cheri Merz (Editor)

## Back and Neck Pain

**The 15 Minute Back Pain and Neck Pain Management Program:** Back Pain and Neck Pain Treatment and Relief 15 Minutes a Day No Surgery No Drugs. Effective, Quick and Lasting Back and Neck Pain Relief. John McArthur (Author)

## Arthritis

**Arthritis:** Arthritis Relief for Osteoarthritis, Rheumatoid Arthritis, Gout, Psoriatic Arthritis, and Juvenile Arthritis. Follow The Arthritis Diet, Cure and Treatment Free Yourself From The Pain. John McArthur (Author)

## Depression

**How to Break the Grip of Depression:** Read How Robert Declared War On Depression ... And Beat It! John McArthur (Author)

## Pregnancy

**Pregnancy Nutrition:** Pregnancy Food. Pregnancy Recipes. Healthy Pregnancy Diet. Pregnancy Health. Pregnancy Eating and Recipes. Nutritional Tips and 63 Delicious Recipes for Moms-to-Be. Corinne Watson (Author), John McArthur (Author)

**Pregnancy and Childbirth:** Expecting a Baby. Pregnancy Guide. Pregnancy What to Expect. Pregnancy Health. Pregnancy Eating and Recipes. Cheri Merz (Author), John McArthur (Author)

## Allergies

**Allergy Free:** Fast Effective Drug-free Relief for Allergies. Allergy Diet. Allergy Treatments. Allergy Remedies. Natural Allergy Relief. John McArthur (Author), Cheri Merz (Editor)